CONTENTS

Yogatattva Upanishad

Belonging to Krishna Yajurveda

Vedantic View on the Truth of Yoga

(English Translation Accompanied by Sanskrit Text in Roman Transliteration)

Translated into English by
Swami Vishnuswaroop

Divine Yoga Institute
Kathmandu, Nepal

ALSO BY THE AUTHOR

Yoga Kundalini Upanishad (in English)
Yoga Darshana Upanishad (in English)
Minor Yoga Upanishads (in English)
HathaYoga Pradipika (in English)
Triyoga Upanishad (in English)
Gheranda Samhita (in English)
Goraksha Samhita (in English)
Triyoga Samhita (in English)
Shiva Samhita (in English)
Shiva Samhita (in Nepali)
Surya Namskara (in Nepali)
Durga Strotram (in Nepali)
Vagalamukhi Stotram (in Nepali)
Amogha Shivakavacham (in Nepali)

ISBN: 9781521780299

DEDICATION

Tasmai Shri Gurave Namah!

This book is dedicated to my Guru Swami Satyananda Saraswati,
The Founder of Bihar School of Yoga, Munger, India.

SALUATATION TO GURU

First of all I would like to express my heartfelt salutations to Adinatha (the Primordial Master) and my Guru for their unwavering inspiration and guidance I have received for my work. I realize that my firm faith and belief in God and Guru is a motivational gift for me in completing this work. I could never have done it without their blessings.

I am always thankful to Ms. Bhawani Uprety for her untiring support she has provided me during my involvement in writing and translating various classical texts on yoga. My due thanks goes to her forever.

On the occasion of the Guru Purnima Day I wish that may God and Guru inspire us to tread the path of yoga in order to achieve the ultimate goal of human life!

- Swami Vishnuswaroop
Guru Purnima, 2017

INTRODUCTION

This *Upaniśad* belongs to *Kriśna Yajurveda.* The various subject matters of yoga are elaborately described in it. In the beginning Lord *Viśnu* imparts the knowledge of the mysterious truth of yoga to Brahma. It is said that yoga is a means to attain the highest state or self-realization. *Mantra Yoga, Laya Yoga, Haṭha Yoga* and *Rāja Yoga* and their four states – *ārambha, ghaṭa, paricaya* and *niśpatti* are described. Further the moderation in diet and daily routine for a yogi are stated. The description of preliminary signs of *yoga siddhis* (perfection in yoga) and instructions for keeping oneself away from these powers are detailed.

Yoga *Sādhanā* when followed and practiced with full devotion and a concentrated mind certainly bestows success to a yogi and he is equipped with all the *siddhis* (*aṇimā*, *garimā* and *mahimā*, etc.). He becomes the authority of the divine powers. Finally, after realizing the essence of the Self like an unwavering lamp within himself, he is liberated from the worldly cycles of death and birth.

Thus, the major subjects of yoga with its with its ultimate goal are presented in this *Upaniṣad*, which makes it unique and complete.

A key to transliteration is given at the end of the text. It is hoped that this book will be helpful for all who are interested to understand the *vedantic* view on the truth of yoga.

Publisher

YOGATATTVA UPANISHAD

Śānti Pāṭha

om sahanāvavatu.

saha nau bhunaktu.

saha viryam karavāvahai.

tejasvināvadhītamastu mā vidviśāvahai.

om śāntiḥ om śāntiḥ om śāntiḥ!

Om. May He protect both of us together. May He nourish both of us together. May both of us get strength and power together. May our knowledge (given and received between us) be powerful. May there be no animosity between us. Om. May there be peace, peace and peace again in all three worlds and May the three types of pains/miseries be peaceful.

Description of Yogatattva

yogatattvaṃ pravakśyāmi yogināṃ hitakāmyayā /

yacchrutvā ca paṭhitvā ca sarvapāpaiḥ pramuchyate //1//

Now I am going to describe *yogatattva* (truth of yoga) for the benefit and fulfillment of the desire of yogis. All sins are destroyed by hearing and studying about it. – 1.

Mahāyogī Viṣṇu

viṣṇurnāma mahāyogī mahābhūto mahātapāḥ /

tattvamārge yathā dīpo dṛśyate puruṣottamaḥ //2//

Puruṣottama (the Supreme Personality) called *Viṣṇu* is *Mahāyogī* (the Supreme Yogi), *Mahābhūta* (the Supreme Being and *Mahātapas* (the Supreme Ascetic)). He is luminous like a lamp on the path of the truth. – 2.

tamārādhya jagannātham praṇipatya pitāmahaḥ /

papraccha yogatattvam me brūhi cāṣṭāṅgasamyutam //3//

Pitāmaha (the Grandfather) *Brahmā* having duly worshipped and saluted *Jagannātha* (the Lord of the universe, *Viṣṇu*) asked Him, "O Lord! Please explain me *yogatattva* (the truth of yoga) with its eight limbs. -3.

Net of Māyā

tamuvāca hṛṣīkeśo vakśyāmi śruṇu tattvataḥ /

sarve jīvāḥ sukhairdhuḥkhairmāyājālena veṣṭitāḥ //4//

Having heard this *Hṛṣīkeśa* (Lord *Viṣṇu*) replied, "I explain the truth (of yoga) in essence. Listen it carefully. All souls are entrapped in the net of happiness and sorrow of *Māyā* (illusion). -4.

teṣāṃ muktikaraṃ margaṃ māyājālanikṛntanam /

janmamṛtyujarā vyādhināśanaṃ mṛtyutārakam //5//

It is the path which gives liberation by destroying the net of *Māyā*. It is the destroyer of birth and death, old age and disease. It is the conqueror of death. -5.

Kaivalya Pada

nānāmārgaistu duṣprāpaṃ kaivalyaṃ paramaṃ padam /

patitāḥ śāstrajāleṣu prajñayā tena mohitā //6//

It is difficult to attain *kaivalya pada* (the Supreme State) following various paths. The wise men fall into net of various *śāstras* (scriptutes) and their minds are deluded by the knowledge (of those *śāstras*). -6.

anirvācyaṃ padaṃ vaktuṃ na śakyaṃ taiḥ surairapi /

svātmaprakāśarūpaṃ tatkiṃ śāstreṇa prakāsyate //7//

That Indefinable State cannot be described even by the gods. One which is in the form of self-shining *Ātma,* how can It be clarified by the *śāstras*? -7.

niṣkalaṃ nirmalaṃ śāntaṃ sarvātītaṃ nirāmayam /

tadeva jīvarūpeṇa puṇyapāpaphalairvṛtam //8//

He is undivided, without taints, tranquil, beyond all and free from diseases. It is in the form of *Jīva* becomes complete by the results of (its) virtue and sin. -8.

Paramātman Beyond All

paramātmapadaṃ nityaṃ tatkathaṃ jīvatāṃ gatam /

sarvabhāvapadātītaṃ jñānarūpaṃ nirañjanam //9//

When the seat of *Paramātman* is eternal, above and beyond all the state of all existence in the form of wisdom and free from any stains, how does it become *Jīva*? -9.

Creation of Piṇḍa

vārivatsphuritaṃ tasminstatrāhaṃkṛtirutthitā /

pañcātmakamabhūtpiṇḍaṃ dhātubaddaṃ guṇātmakam //10//

In His Spirit there arose a bubble like in water and there appeared *ahaṃkāra* (ego). From it there appeared a *piṇḍa* (body) made of *pañcabhūta* (the five elements) bound together with *dhātus* and *guṇas.* -10.

sukhaduḥkhaiḥ samāyuktaṃ jīvabhāvanayā kuru /

tena jīvābhidhā proktā viśuddhaiḥ paramātmani //11//

The *Pure Paramātman* associating with happiness and misery thought to take the form of *jīva.* Due to this reason, it was called *jīva.* -11.

kāmakrodhabhayaṃ cāpi mohalobhamado rajaḥ /

janma mṛtyuśca kārpaṇyaṃ śokastandrā kśudhā tṛṣā //12//

tṛṣnā lajjā bhayaṃ duḥkhaṃ viṣādo harśa eva ca /

ebhirdoṣairvinirmuktaḥ sa jīvaḥ kevalo mataḥ //13//

The *jīva* is regarded to be *kevala* (pure) when it is freed from these faults of passion, anger, fear, delusion, greed, pride, lust, birth, death, avarice, grief, torpor, hunger, thirst, craving, shame, terror, pain, grief and cheer. -12-13.

Importance of Knowledge and Yoga

tasmāddoṣavināśārthamupāyaṃ kathayāmi te /

yogahīnaṃ kathaṃ jñānaṃ mokśadaṃ bhavati dhruvam //14//

yogohi jñānahīnastu na kśamo mokśakarmaṇi /

tasmājjñānaṃ ca yogaṃ ca mumukśudṛdhamabhyaset //15//

Therefore, I shall describe you the measures to destroy those faults (mentioned above). How the knowledge without yoga can certainly give liberation? Yoga without knowledge also cannot attain liberation. Hence, one who wishes for attaining liberation should firmly practice both the knowledge and yoga. -14-15.

The World After Ajñāna

ajñānādeva saṃsāro jñānādeva vimucyate /

jñānasvarūpamevādau jñānaṃ jñeyaikasādhanam //16//

The worldly existence certainly appears from *ajñāna* (ignorance). One is certainly liberated from it through *jñāna* (knowledge) alone. In the beginning knowledge alone exists. So, the knowledge alone is the means to achieve *jñeya* (what ought to be known). -16.

Nature of Saccidānanda

jñātaṃ yena nijaṃ rūpaṃ kaivalyaṃ paramaṃ padam /

niṣkalaṃ nirmalaṃ sākśātsaccidānandarūpakaṃ //17//

utpattisthitisaṃhārasphūrtijñānavivarjitam /

etajjñānamiti proktamatha yogaṃ bravīmi te //18//

By which one knows his true form and the highest state which is pure in the form *Saccidānanda* (Truth, Existence and Bliss), free from fault, creation, existence, destruction and appearance is the real *jñāna.* Now I describe you about yoga. -17-18.

Types of Yoga

yogo hi bahudhā brahmanbhidyate vyavahārataḥ /

mantrayogo layaścaiva haṭho'sau rājayogataḥ //19//

O *Brahman*! Various types of yoga has been described according to its usage, e.g. *Mantra Yoga, Laya Yoga, Haṭha Yoga, Rāja Yoga,* etc. -19.

Stages of Yoga

ārambhaśca ghaṭaścaiva tathā paricayaḥ smṛtaḥ /

niṣpattiścetyavasthā ca sarvatra parikīrtitā //20//

Four stages of yoga has been described everywhere. These stages are *ārambha, ghaṭa, paricaya* and *niṣpatti.* -20.

Characteristics of Stages

eteṣāṃ lakśaṇaṃ brahmanvavakśye śṛuṇu samāsataḥ /

mātṛkādiyutaṃ mantraṃ dvādaśābdaṃ tu yo japet //21//

krameṇa labhate jñānamaṇimādiguṇānvitaṃ /

alpabuddhirimaṃ yogaṃ sevate sādhakādhamaḥ //22//

Listen, O *Brahman*! I shall describe you the characteristics of these (stages) briefly. One who practices a *mantra* along with its *mātṛkā* (proper intonations of the sounds) for twelve years; he then gradually obtains the wisdom of *aṇimā siddhi*, etc. But this type of yoga is practiced by those people who have low level of intellect and they are low class *sādhakas*. -21-22.

layayogaścittalayaḥ kotiśaḥ parikīrtitaḥ /

gacchantiṣṭhansvapanbhuñjandhyāyenniṣkalamīśvaram //23//

The absorption of *chitta* (the mind) is *Laya Yoga*. It has been described having millions types. One should constantly contemplate the undivided *Īśvara* while walking, sitting, sleeping and eating. -23.

sa eva layayogaḥ syāddhaṭhayogamataḥ śruṇu /

yamaśca niyamaścaiva āsanaṃ prāṇasamyamaḥ //24//

pratyāhāro dhāraṇā ca dhyānaṃ bhrūmadhyame harim /

samādhiḥ samatāvasthā sāṣṭāṅgo yoga ucyate //25//

It is *Laya Yoga* that has been described above. Now listen about *Haṭha Yoga*. *Yama* (forbearance), *niyama* (religious observance), āsana (posture), *prāṇasamyama* (control of breath), *pratyāhāra* (withdrawal of the senses), *dhāraṇā* (concentration), *dhyāna* (meditation) on *Hari* in the middle of the eyebrows and *samādhi* (superconcious state) or *samatāvasthā* (the equilibrium state of mind) are called the *Aṣṭāṅga* Yoga. -24-25.

Various Mudrās

mahāmudrā mahābandho mahāvedhaśca khecari /

jālandharoḍḍiyāṇaśca mūlabandhastathaiva ca //26//

dīrghapraṇavasandhānaṃ siddhāntaśravaṇaṃ param /

vajroli cāmarolī ca sahajolī tridhā matā //27//

Mahāmudrā, *mahābandha*, *mahāvedha* and *khecari*, *jālandhara bandha*, *uḍḍiyāṇa bandha*, *mūlabandha*, *dīrgha praṇava sandhāna* (constant repetition of long *AUM* without interruption), hearing of the ultimate reality and the three *vajroli*, *amarolī* and *sahajolī* are called *mudrās*. -26-27.

Yama, Niyama and Āsana

eteṣāṃ lakśaṇaṃ brahmanpratyekaṃ śruṇu tattvataḥ /

ladhvāhāro yameṣveko mukhyo bhavati netaraḥ //28//

ahiṃsā niyameṣvekā mukhyā vai caturānana /

siddhaṃ padmaṃ tathā śiṃhaṃ bhadraṃ ceti catuṣṭayam //29//

O *Brahman!* Now hear the characteristics of each of them in essence. Of *yamas*, eating or taking little food is main thing and *ahiṃsā* (non-violence) is prime in *niyama*. *Siddha, padma, śiṃha* and *bhadra* are the main four postures. -28-29.

Obstacles in Yoga Practice

prathamābhyāsakāle tu vighnāḥ syuścaturānana /

ālasyaṃ katthanaṃ dhūrtagoṣṭhī mantrādisādhanaṃ //30//

O *Caturānana* (Four-faced One) first of all in the preliminary stage of practice these obstacles arise, e.g. laziness, self-praise, meeting with cunning people, practice of mantras, etc. -31.

dhātustrilaulyakādīni mṛgatṛṣṇāmayāni vai /

jñātvā sudhīstyajetsarvān vighnānpuṇyaprabhāvataḥ //31//

A wise practitioner should consider metals (coin, gold, silver etc. wealth), woman, restlessness, etc. in the form of mirage and obstacles and abandon them by the power of his virtuous deeds. -31.

All About a Maṭha

praṇāyāmaṃ tataḥ kuryātpadmāsanagataḥ svayam /

suśobhanaṃ maṭhaṃ kuryātsūkśmadvāraṃ tu nirvraṇam //32//

Then performing *padmāsana*, he should practice *praṇāyāma*. He should build a beautiful *maṭha* (hut, cottage, cell) with a small door and without any holes. -32.

suṣṭhu liptaṃ gomayena sudhayā vā prayatnataḥ /

maṭkuṇairmaśakairlūtairvarjitaṃ ca prayatnataḥ //33//

Then it should be smeared well with cow-dung and cleaned properly. With due care, it should be made free from bugs, mosquitoes, spiders, etc. -33.

dine dine ca saṃmṛṣṭaṃ saṃmārjanyā viśeṣataḥ /

yāsitaṃ ca sugandhena dhūpitaṃ guggulādibhiḥ //34//

It should be specially cleaned well every day. It should be scented with good incense and smoked with *guggula* (fragrant gum). -34.

nātyucchritaṃ nātīnicaṃ cailājinakuśottaram /

tatropaviśya medhāvī padmāsanasamanvitaḥ //35//

Sitting on a seat neither too high nor too low which is made of either cloth (cotton), deerskin or *kuśa* (the sacred grass), the wise practitioner should perform the *padmāsana.* -35.

Practice of Prāṇāyāma

ṛjukāyaḥ prañjaliśca praṇamediṣṭadevatām /

tato dakśiṇahastasya aṅguṣṭhenaiva piṅgalām //36//

nirudhya pūrayedvāyumiḍayā tu śanaiḥ śanaiḥ /

yathāśaktyavirodhena tataḥ kuryācca kumbhakam //37//

Keeping his body straight and joining the hands together, he should salute his *iṣṭa devatā* (favorite deity). Then closing *piṅgalā* (the right nostril) with his right thumb, he should slowly inhale through *iḍā* (the left nostril) and perform *kumbhaka* (retention of breath) according to his capacity.

punastyajetpiṅgalayā śanaireva na vegataḥ /

punaḥ piṅgalāpurya pūraedudaraṃ śanaiḥ //38//

dhārayitvā yothāśakti recayediḍayā śanaiḥ /

yathā tyajettayāpūrya dhārayedavirodhata //39//

Then he should exhale slowly, not fast through the right nostril. Then he should slowly fill his stomach through the right nostril and retain the breath inside according to his capacity and then exhale it slowly through the left nostril. Whichever nostril is used for exhalation, the air should be inhaled through the same nostril; it should be retained according to one's capacity and exhaled through the opposite nostril. In this way, one should go on practicing it in a sequential order without break. -38-39.

About the Mātrā (Time Measure)

jānu pradakśiṇīkṛtya na drutaṃ na vilambitam /

aṅgulisphoṭanaṃ kuryātsā mātrā parigīyate //40//

Neither very speedily nor very slowly, one should complete circle of the knee with the palm of the hand and snap the fingers (usually the thumb and middle finger) once. The time (length for doing so) is called a *mātrā*. -40.

iḍayā vāyumāropya śanaiḥ ṣoḍaśamātrayā /

kumbhayetpūritaṃ paścāccatuḥṣaṣṭyā tu mātrayā //41//

recayetpiṅgalānāḍyā dvātriṃśanmātrayā punaḥ /

punaḥ piṅgalayāpūrya purvavatsusamāhitaḥ //42//

One should inhale the air through the left nostril for sixteen *mātrās* and then retain it (inside) for sixty-four *mātrās* and exhale the air through the right nostril for thirty-two *mātrās*. Again he should inhale through the right nostril and continue the practice as before. -41-42.

Time of Prāṇāyāma Practice

prātarmadhyaṃdine sāyamardharātre ca kumbhakān /

śanairaśītiparyantaṃ caturvāraṃ samabyaset //43//

One should practice the *kumbhakas* (retention of breath) in the morning, at noon, in the evening and midnight four times a day, slowly and slowly extending the numbers of *kumbhakas* up to eighty. -43.

Purification of Nāḍīs

evam māsatrayābhyāsānnāḍīśuddhistato bhavet /

yadā tu nāḍīśuddhiḥ syāttadā cinhāni bāhyataḥ //44//

In this way, by the practice of three months the *nāḍīs* are purified. When the *nāḍīs* have been purified, then external signs are seen (on the physical level). -44.

Result of Nāḍī Purification

jāyante yogino dehe tāni vakśyāmyaśeṣataḥ /

śarīralaghutā dīptirjāṭharāgnivivardhanam //45//

kṛśatvaṃ ca śarīrasya tadā jāyate niścitam /

yogavighnakarāhāraṃ varjayedyogavittamaḥ //46//

I shall describe all the external signs which are: lightness of the body, shiny tone (of the body), strengthening of digestive fire and slimness of the body. The excellent yogi should give up those foods that are harmful to yoga practice. -46.

Prohibition of Foods

lavaṇaṃ sarṣapaṃ cāmlamuṣṇam rūkśaṃ ca tīkśṇakam /

śākajātaṃ rāmaṭhādi vanhistripathasevanam //47//

prātaḥ snānopavāsādikāyakleśāṃśca varjayet /

abhyāsakāle prathamaṃ śastaṃ kśīrājyabhojanam //48//

Salt, oil (mustard) sour, hot, pungent, or green vegetables; spices like asafoetida, etc., sitting near fire, (association with) women, walking, early morning bath, fasting, etc. should be given up. In the preliminary stage of practice, food made of the mixture of milk and ghee is excellent. -47-48.

Yogic Food

godhūmamudgaśālyannaṃ yogavṛddhikaraṃ viduḥ /

tataḥ paraṃ yatheṣṭaṃ tu śaktaḥ syādvāyudhāraṇe //49//

Foods that are made of wheat, lentil and rice are said to promote the practice of yoga. By practicing in this way, the yogi gains the ability for holding the breath as long as according to his will. -49.

Kevala Kumbhaka

yatheṣṭadhāraṇādvāyoḥ sidhyetkevalakumbhakaḥ /

kevale kumbhake siddhe recapūravivarjite //50//

After gaining the ability to retain the breath as long as comfortable, perfection in '*kevala kumbhaka*' (spontaneous retention of breath) is achieved. Then inhalation and exhalation should be given up. -50.

Result of Kevala Kumbhaka

na tasya durlabhaṃ kiñcittriṣu lokeṣu vidyate /

prasvedo jāyate pūrvaṃ mardanaṃ tena kārayet //51//

After having done it (mentioned above), there is nothing unachievable for him in all the three worlds. When there is sweating during the practice, it should be rubbed on the body. -51.

tato'pi dhāraṇādvāyoḥ krameṇaiva śanaiḥ śanaiḥ /

kampo bhavati dehasya āsanasthasya dehinaḥ //52//

When the ability of retaining the breath increases very slowly, in its interval, the body of the yogi seated in his āsana starts to tremble. -52.

tato'dhikatarābhyāsāddārdurī svena jāyate /

yathā ca darduro bhāva utplutyotplutya gacchati //53//

padmāsanasthito yogī tathā gacchati bhūtale /

tato'dhikatarābhyāsādbhūmityāgaśca jāyate //54//

Then practicing furthermore, the attempts made by a yogi are similar to a frog. Like the frog jumps off and comes back to the ground, so is the condition of the yogi sitting in *padmāsana.* When the practice is increased further, he starts to rise above the ground. -53-54.

Levitation of the Yogi

padmāsanastha evāsau bhūmimutsṛjyavartate /

atimānuṣaceṣṭādi tathā sāmarthyamudbhavet //55//

The yogi seated in *padmāsana*, due to his advanced practice remains rising in the air. In this way, he gains the power to perform superhuman acts. -55.

No Demo of Powers

na darśayecca sāmarthyaṃ darśanaṃ vīryavattaram /

svalpaṃ vā bahudhā duḥkhaṃ yogī na vyathate tadā //56//

A yogi should not demonstrate his power and ability to others. Seeing in himself (his power and ability), he should promote his enthusiasm. Then he is not troubled by any minor or major pain. -57.

Decrease of Bodily Discharge

alpamūtrapurīṣaśca svalpanidraśca jāyate /

kīlavo dūṣikā lālā svedadurgandhatānete // 57//

etāni sarvathā tasya na jāyante tataḥ param /

tato'dhikatarābhyāsādbalamutpadhyate bahu //58//

The yogi's urine, defecation and sleep are decreased. He will not have eye and nasal discharges, also there will be not be any sweat (in his body), saliva and bad smell in his mouth. By continuing his practice further, he attains great power. -57-58.

Bhūcara Siddhi

yena bhūcarasiddhiḥ syādbhūcaraṇām jaye kśamaḥ /

vyāghro vā śarabho vāpi gajo gavaya eva vā //59//

siṃho vā yoginā tena mṛyante hastatāḍitāḥ /

kandarpasya yathā rūpaṃ tathā syādapi yoginaḥ //60//

By this (power) the yogi achieves *bhūcara siddhi*, which bestows him victory over all the creatures in this earth. Tiger, *śarabha* (a kind of deer), elephant, wild bull or lion are killed by the blow of his hand. The appearance of the yogi becomes beautiful similar to *kandarpa* (the god of love). -59-60.

tadrūpavaśagā nāryaḥ kāṅkśante tasya saṅgamam /

yadi saṅgaṃ karotyeṣa tasya bindukśayo bhavet //61//

Being infatuated by the beautiful appearance of the yogi, women desire to enjoy his association with them. If he fulfills their desire, his semen will be destroyed. -61.

Preservation of Bindu

varjayitvā striyāḥ saṅgaṃ kuryādabhyāsamādarāt /

yogino'ṅge sugandhaśca jāyate bindudhāraṇāt //62//

Therefore, giving up the association of women, he should go in doing his practice with reverence. By the preservation of *bindu* (semen), the body of the yogi emits fragrance. -62.

Practice of Praṇava

tato rahasyupāviṣṭaḥ praṇavaṃ plutamātrayā /

japetpūrvārjitānāṃ tu pāpānāṃ nāśahetave //63//

Then staying in a secret place, he should go on repeating *praṇava* (*AUM* or *OM*) with *plutamātrā* (the three *mātrās* in which the intonation is prolonged) in order to destroy all his sins of the past lives. -63.

Ārambha Avasthā

sarvavighnaharo mantraḥ praṇavaḥ sarvadoṣahā /

evamabhyāsayogena siddhirārambhasaṃbhavā //64//

The mantra *praṇava* is the destroyer of all obstacles and impurities. By this yogic practice he can achieve the perfection of *ārambha* (first or beginning) *avasthā* (stage). -64.

Ghaṭa Avasthā

tato bhavedghaṭāvasthā pavanabhyāsatatparā /

prāṇo'pāno mano buddhirjīvātmaparamātmanoḥ //65//

anyonyasyāvirodhena ekatā ghaṭate yadā /

ghaṭāvastheti sā proktā taccinhāni bravīmyaham //66//

After this *ghaṭa avasthā* is attained by intently practicing the retention of breath. By the practice through which when the perfect union is established without any contradiction between *prāṇa* and *apāna*, *mana* and *buddhi*, *jīvātmā* and *paramātmā* is called *ghaṭa avasthā.* I am going to describe its signs. -65-66.

Signs of Ghaṭa Avasthā

pūrva yaḥ kathito'bhyāsaścaturthāṃśaṃ parigrahet /

divā vā yadi vā sāyaṃ yāmamātraṃ samabhyaset //67//

ekavāraṃ pratidinaṃ kuryātkevalakumbhakam /

indriyāṇīndriyārthebhyo yatpratyāharaṇaṃ sphuṭam //68//

yogī kumbhakamāsthāya pratyāhāraḥ sa ucyate /

yadyatpaśyati cakśurbhyāṃ tattadātmeti bhāvayet //69//

Whatever time period for his practice was mentioned before, now he should only practice one-fourth of the specified time. Whether it is during the day or during the night, he should practice only for a *yāma* (three hours). He should practice *kevala kumbhaka* only once a day. *Pratyāhāra* occurs when the senses are withdrawn from their respective sense-organs/objects. When a yogi is established in *kumbhaka*, it is called *pratyāhāra*. At that time whatever the yogi sees through his eyes, he should regard it as *Ātman*. -67-69.

yadyacchṛṇoti karṇābhyāṃ tattadātmeti bhāvayet /

labhate nāsayā yadhyattattadātmeti bhāvayet //70//

Whatever he hears with his ears, he should regard it as *Ātman*. Whatever he smells through his noses, with his skin, he should regard it as *Ātman*. -70.

Regarding Everything As Ātman

jihvayā yadrasaṃ hyatti tattadādmeti bhāvayet /

tvacā yadyatspṛśedyogī tattadātmeti bhāvayet //71//

Whatever he tastes with his tongue, he should regard it as *Ātman*. Whatever the yogi touches with his skin, he should regard it as *Ātman*. -71.

evaṃ jñānendriyāṇāṃ tu tattadātmani dhārayet /

yāmamātraṃ pratidinaṃ yogī yatnādatandritaḥ //72//

In this way, whatever objects of senses are there, the yogi should hold them in his Inner Self and he should practice it every day with due effort for one *yama* (three hours). -72.

Achievement of Various Siddhis

yathā vā cittasāmarthyaṃ jāyate yogino dhruvam /

dūraśrutirdūradṛṣṭiḥ kśaṇāddūrāgamastathā //73//

vāksiddhiḥ kāmarūpatvamadṛśyakaraṇī tathā /

malamūtrapralepena lohādeḥ svarṇatā bhavet //74//

khe gatistasya jāyeta santatābhyāsayogataḥ /

sadā buddhimatā bhāvyaṃ yoginā yogasiddhaye //75//

Thus, when the mental power of the yogi is certainly increased through practice, then various *siddhis* (supernatural powers) are gained by the yogi like clairaudience, clairvoyance, ability to go anywhere in a moment, perfection of speech, ability to take any form as desired, ability to become invisible and transformation of iron into gold by smearing his excretion (on iron), ability to travel through space. The wise yogi should always contemplate on *yoga siddhi* (perfection of yoga i.e. union with *Paramātman*). -73-75.

Concealment of Siddhis

ete vighnā mahāsiddherna ramettesu buddhimān /

na darśayetsvasāmarthyaṃ yasya kasyāpi yogirāṭ //76//

The wise yogi should not be delighted with all these great powers. The sovereign yogi should never disclose and demonstrate his powers to anyone. -76.

yathā mūḍho yathā mūrkho yathā badhira eva vā /

tathā varteta lokasya svasāmarthyasya guptaye //77//

Therefore, the yogi should remain as an ignorant, foolish or deaf person among the people in general. He should conceal his abilities and be in secret. -77.

śiṣyāśca svasvakāryeṣu prārthayanti na saṃśayaḥ /

tattaṭkarmakaravyagraḥ svābhyāse'vismṛto bhavet //78//

The disciples of the yogi certainly request him for his involvement in their desired karmas (activities). But the yogi should never be away/forget his own practice being engrossed in others' activities. -78.

Devotion to Yogic Practice

sarvavyāpāramutsṛjya yoganiṣṭho bhavedyatiḥ /

avismṛtya gurorvākyamabhyasettadaharniśam //79//

He should give up all other activities and devote himself to the practice of yoga. Without forgetting the words of his Guru, he should constantly practice day and night. -79.

Ghaṭa Avasthā

evaṃ bhavedghaṭāvasthā santatābhyāsayogataḥ /

anabhyāsavataścaiva vṛthāgoṣṭhyā na siddhyati //80//

In this way, he attains *ghaṭāvasthā* through his continuous involvement in his yogic practice. Perfection is attained through constant practice, not by mere gossip. -80

Paricaya Avasthā

tasmātsarvaprayatnena yogameva sadābhyaset /

tataḥ paricayāvasthā jāyate'bhyāsayogataḥ //81//

vāyuḥ paricito yatnādagninā saha kuṇḍalīm /

bhāvayitvā suṣumnāyāṃ praviśedanirodhataḥ //82//

Therefore, the yogi should always go on practicing with all efforts. Then, there occurs an auspicious beginning of *paricaya avasthā* by the practice of yoga. For (achieving) this stage, visualizing the *kuṇḍalinī* along with the *agni* (fire) fired by the *vāyu* should be made to enter the *suṣumnā* through the practice without any disturbance. -81-82.

Mind to Mahā Patha

vāyunā saha cittaṃ ca praviśecca mahāpatham /

yasya cittaṃ svapavanaṃ suṣumnāṃ praviśediha //83//

bhūmirāpo'nalo vāyurākāśaśceti paṇcakaḥ /

yeṣu pañcasu devānāṃ dhāraṇā pañcadhocyate //84//

Then *chitta* (the mind) along with the *vāyu* should be directed to *mahā patha* (the great path i.e. *suṣumnā*). Here (if) one's mind along with the *vāyu* entered *suṣumnā* (the middle psychic pathway), then he should contemplate on five deities in the form of the five elements – *bhūmi* (earth), *āpa* (water) *anala* (fire), *vāyu* (air) and *ākāśa* (ether). These five *dhāraṇās* are called *pañca dhāraṇā* (concentration on the five elements). -83-84.

Practice of Pañca Dhāraṇā

pādādijānuparyantaṃ pṛthivīsthānamucyate /

pṛthivi caturastraṃ ca pītavarṇaṃ lavarṇakam //85//

pārthive vāyumāropya lakāreṇa samanvitam /

dhyāyaścaturbhujākāraṃ caturvaktraṃ hiraṇmayam //86//

It is said that the area of *pṛthivī tattva* is from the feet to the knees. It has four-sided shape, is of yellow color and its *varṇa* (alphabet) '*la*'. Placing the *vāyu* upon the earth element in combination with the '*lakāra*' (the alphabet '*la*'), one should contemplate there on golden colored *brahmā* having four arms and four mouths. -85-86.

Dhāraṇā on Pṛthivī Tattva

dhārayetpaṇca ghaṭikāḥ pṛthivījayamāpnuyāt /

prithivīyogato mṛtyurna bhavedasya yoginaḥ //87//

In this way, by concentrating there for *paṇca ghaṭikā* (two hours) he gains victory over the earth element. Such a yogi does not face his death due to his contact with the earth (i.e. he cannot be stroked and killed by the earth). -87.

Dhāraṇā on Āpas Tattva

ājānoḥ pāyuparyantamapāṃ sthānaṃ prakīrtitam /

āpo'rdhacandraṃ śuklaṃ ca vaṃbījaṃ parikīrtitam //88//

vāruṇe vāyumāropya vakāreṇa samanvitam /

smarannārāyaṇaṃ devaṃ caturbāhuṃ kirīṭinam //89//

śuddhaspahṭikasaṅkāśaṃ pītavāsasamacyutam /

dhārayetpaṇca ghaṭikāḥ sarvapāpaiḥ pramucyate //90//

It is said that the area of *āpas tattva* is from the knees to the anus. It has a crescent shape, is of white color and '*vaṃ*' is its *bīja*. Placing the *vāyu* upon the earth element in combination with the *bīja* '*vaṃ*', one should contemplate there on the God *Nārāyaṇa* who has four arms, is wearing a crown, is pure like crystal in his orange clothes and is non-decaying. By practicing this *dhāraṇā* there for *paṇca ghaṭikā* (two hours), he is freed from all sins. -88-90.

Dhāraṇā on Agni Tattva

tato jalādbhayaṃ nāsti jale mṛtyurna vidyate /

āpāyorhṛdayāntaṃ ca vanhisthānaṃ prakīrtitam //91//

Then there is no fear from water for him and he does not face his death due to water. It is said that *vanhi sthāna* (the place of fire) is from *āpas tattva* (the area of anus) to *hṛdaya* (the heart). -91.

vanhistrikoṇaṃ raktaṃ ca rephākśarasamudbhavam /

vanhau cānilamāropya rephākśarasamujjvalam //92//

Agni is of triangular shape. Its color is red and it is originated with *repha akśara* (the alphabet '*ra*'). Placing the *vāyu* upon the fire element the radiant alphabet '*ra*' should be combined there.

Contemplation on Triyakśa

triyakśaṃ varadaṃ rudraṃ taruṇāditya sannibham /

bhasmodhūlitasarvāṅgaṃ suprasannamanusmaran //93//

One should always contemplate with a very happy mind on *Rudra*, the three-eyed one, who fulfills all wishes, who has the color of the rising sun and who has smeared ashes all over his body. -93.

Result of Triyakśa Dhāraṇā

dhārayetpañca ghatikā vanhināsau na dāhyate /

na dahyate śarīraṃ ca praviṣṭasyāgnimaṇḍale //94//

By practicing this *dhāraṇā* there for *paṇca ghaṭikā* (two hours), he is not burnt by the fire. Besides, his body does not burn even by chance fallen in *āgni maṇḍala* (the sphere of the burning fire). -94.

Dhāraṇā Vāyu Tattva

āhṛdayādbhruvormadyaṃ vāyusthānaṃ prakīrtitam /

vāyuḥṣaṭkoṇakaṃ kṛṣṇaṃ yakārākśarabhāsuram //95//

It is said that the area of *vāyu sthāna* (the place of air) is from the heart to the middle of the eyebrows. It is of hexagonal shape, has black color and is radiant with *yakāra akśara* (the alphabet '*ya*'). -95.

Dhāraṇā on the Īśvara

mārutaṃ marutāṃ sthāne yakārākśarabhāsuram /

dhārayettatra sarvajñamīśvaraṃ viśvatomukham //96//

Placing the *vāyu* upon its own place (the area of *vāyu tattva*) in combination with the radiant *yakāra akśara* (the alphabet '*ya*'), one should contemplate there on the *Īśvara,* the Omniscient and *Viśvatomukha* (one who is facing everywhere). -96.

Result of the Īśvara Dhāraṇā

dhārayetpañca ghaṭikā vāyuvadvyomago bhavet /

maraṇaṃ na tu vāyośca bhayaṃ bhavati yoginaḥ //97//

By practicing this *dhāraṇā* there (on *Viśvatomukha*) for *paṇca ghaṭikā* (two hours), he can go to the space like the air. The yogi does not die and have any fear from the air. -97.

Dhāraṇā on Ākāśa Tattva

āṃbhrūmadhyāttu mūrdhāntamākāśasthānamuccyate /

vyoma vṛttaṃ ca dhūmraṃ ca hakārākśarabhāsuram //98//

It is said that the area of *ākāśa sthāna* (the place of ether) is from the middle of the eyebrows to the top of the head. Its shape is circular like *vyoma vṛtta* (circle of space/sky). It has a smoky color and is radiant with *hakāra akśara* (the alphabet '*ha*'). -98.

Dhāraṇā on Sadāśiva

ākāśe vāyumāropya hakāropari śaṅkaram /

bindurūpaṃ mahādevaṃ vyomakāraṃ sadāśivam //99//

Placing the *vāyu* upon the *ākāśa tattva* (one should concentrate on) *Śaṅkara* above the *hakāra* (the alphabet '*ha*') who is *Mahādeva* in the form of *bindu*. He is *Sadāśiva* (one who is always kind) in the form of *vyoma* (space/sky). -99.

Nature of Lord Śiva

śuddhasphaṭikasaṅkāśaṃ dhṛtabālendumaulinam /

pañcavaktrayutaṃ saumyaṃ daśabāhuṃ trilocanam //100//

The Lord *Śiva* is completely untainted like the pure bright crystal. He is wearing the crescent moon on his head, has five faces, has a pleasant appearance, and has ten hands and three eyes. -100.

Lord Śiva the Cause of All Causes

sarvāyudhairdhṛtākāraṃ sarvabhūṣaṇabhuṣitam /

umārdhadehaṃ varadaṃ sarvakāraṇakāraṇam //101//

The Lord *Śiva* is equipped with all types of arms and decorated with all types of ornaments. Half of his body belongs to *Umā* (*Pārvati*). He is the fulfiller all wishes and is the ultimate source of all causes. -101.

Dhāraṇā on Ākāśa Tattva

ākāśadhāraṇāttasya khecaratvaṃ bhaveddhruvam /

yatra kutra sthito vāpi sukhamatyantamaśnute //102//

By contemplating on Lord *Śiva* in the area of *ākāśa tattva*, certainly the power of going to space/sky is achieved. Through the practice of this *dhāraṇā*, a *sādhaka* may stay anywhere, but he enjoys absolute happiness. -102.

evaṃ ca dhāraṇāh pañca kuryādyogī vicakśaṇaḥ /

tato dṛḍhaśarīraḥ syānmṛtyustasya na vidyate //103//

Thus, the expert yogi should practice these five types of *dhāraṇā*. The body of the yogi becomes very strong due to it and death does not exist for him. -103.

brahmaṇaḥ pralayenāpi na sīdati mahāmatiḥ /

samabhyasettathā dhyānaṃ ghaṭikāṣaṣṭimeva ca /

vāyuṃ nirudhya cākāśe devatāmiṣṭadāmiti //104//

The highly intellect yogi does not die even during the dissolution of the universe by the divine power. He should contemplate on his favorable god who bestows perfection in the area of *ākāśa* for a period of six *ghaṭikās* (2 hours – 24 Minutes) By Stopping The Breath. -104.

Saguṇa and Nirguṇa Dhyāna

saguṇaṃ dhyānametatsyādaṇimādiguṇapradam /

nirguṇadhyānayuktasya samādhiśca tato bhavet //105//

Siddhis like *aṇimādi* (*aṇimā,* etc.) are achieved through the practice of *saguṇa dhyāna* (meditation on gods with attributes or qualities). *Samādhi* is attained through the practice of *nirguṇa dhyāna* (meditation on god devoid of the attributes or qualities). -105

Achievement of Samādhi

dinadvādaśakenaiva samādhiṃ samavāpnuyāt /

vāyuṃ nirudhya medhāvī jīvanmukto bhavatyayam //106//

The exalted yogi attains perfection in *samādhi* in twelve days only. Having retained the *vāyu* (and perfecting the *samādhi*), he accomplishes liberation in his life. -106.

Unity of Jīvātma and Paramātman

samādhiḥ samatāvasthā jīvātmaparamātmanoḥ /

yadi svadehamutsraṣṭumicchā cedutsṛjetsvayam //107//

There is an equal state of *Jīvātma* (Individual Self) and *Paramātman* (Supreme Self) in *Samādhi.* If he wishes to abandon his body, he can do it so of his own accord. -107.

Result of Samādhi

parabrahmaṇi līyate na tasyoṭkrāntiriṣyate /

atha no cetsamutsraṣṭuṃ svasarīraṃ priyaṃ yadi //108//

sarvalokeṣu viharannaṇimādiguṇānvitaḥ /

kadācitsvecchayā devo bhūtvā svarge mahīyate //109//

In this way, the yogi dissolves him into *Parabrahman* and he does not have to be borne again. But if his body is dear to him, he can live in his body and he can go to all the worlds with all *aṇimādi siddhis* (the eight supernatural powers, *aṇimā,* etc.). If he desired, he can become a *devatā* (divine being) at any time and dwell in the heaven. -108-109.

The Yogi's Form As His Wish

manuṣyo vāpi yakśyo vā svecchayāpi kśaṇādbhavet /

simho vyāghro gajo vāśvaḥ svecchayā bahutāmiyat //110//

The yogi can take the form of a human being or a *yakśya* (a supernatural being) at his will. He can also take the form of many animals like a lion, a tiger, an elephant or a horse as per his will. -110.

His Action As His Wish

yatheṣṭameva varteta yadvā yogī maheśvaraḥ /

abhyāsabedato bhedaḥ phalaṃ tu samameva hi //111//

The yogi achieving the position of *Maheśvara*, he can act or behave according to his wishes. The difference is only of the practice; both are certainly equal in view of the result.

Practice of Mahā Bandha

pārṣṇiṃ vāmasya pādasya yonisthāne niyojayet /

prasāryaṃ dakśiṇaṃ pādaṃ hastābhyāṃ dhārayetdṛḍham //112//

One should press the perineum with his left heel and extend the right leg (in the front) and hold it (or its toes) firmly with both hands. -112.

cibukaṃ hṛdi vinyasya pūrayedvāyunā punaḥ /

kumbhakena yathāśakti dhārayitvā tu rechayet //113//

He should place his head on the chest and inhale the air slowly and retain it (inside) as long as possible and then exhale it slowly. -113.

vāmāṅgena samabyasya dakśāṅgena tato'bhyaset /

prasāritastu yaḥ pādastamūrūpari nāmayet //114//

After practicing properly with the left foot, it should be practiced with the right or the perineum should be pressed with leg that was extended before. The leg that was pressing the perineum should be extended and its toes should be grabbed firmly.

ayameva mahābandha ubhayatraivamabhyaset /

mahābandhasthito yogī kṛtvā pūrakamekadhīḥ //115//

vāyunā gatimāvṛtya nibhṛtaṃ kaṇṭhamudrayā /

puṭadvayaṃ samākramya vāyuḥ sphurati satvaram //116//

This is *mahā bandha.* It should be practiced on both sides. The yogi practicing *mahā bandha* with the concentrated mind should inhale the air and reverse the course of the *vāyu* with *kaṇṭha* (throat) *mudrā.* By contracting the both nostrils the *vāyu* is filled up speedily. -115-116.

Practice of Mahāveda

ayameva mahāvedhaḥ siddhairabhyasyate'niśam /

antaḥ kapālakuhare jihvāṃ vyāvṛtya dhārayet //117//

bhrūmadhyadṛṣṭirapyeṣā mudrā bhavati khecarī /

kaṇṭhamākuñcya hṛdaye sthāpayeddṛḍhayā dhiyā //118//

bandho jālandharākyo'yaṃ mṛtyumātaṅgakesarī /

bandho yena suṣumnāyāṃ prāṇastūḍḍīyate yataḥ //119//

uḍyānākhyo hi bandho'yaṃ yogībhiḥ samudāhṛtaḥ /

This is called *mahāvedha. Siddha* yogis always practice it. Inserting the tongue in the cavity of the throat and gazing in the middle of the eyebrows is *khecarī mudrā.* Contracting the neck and placing the head firmly on the chest, this is called the *jālandhara Bandha* which is equal to a lion over the elephant of death. The *Bandha* by which *prāṇa* is raised up through *suṣumnā* is called *uḍḍīyāna bandha* by the yogis. -118-120 (a).

Practice of Yoni Bandha

pārṣṇibhāgena sampīḍya yonimākuñcayeddṛḍham //120//

apānamūrdhvamutthāpya yonibandho'yamucyate /

prāṇapānau nādabindū mūlabandhena caikatām //121//

gatvā yogasya saṃsiddhiṃ yacchato nātra samśayaḥ /

karaṇī viparītākhyā sarvavyādhivināśinī //122//

Pressing the perineum properly by the heel, it should be contracted firmly and then *apāna* should be raised up. This is called to be *yoni bandha. Prāṇa, apāna, nāda* and *bindū* are united through the practice of *mūla bandha.* It bestows perfection in yoga without any doubt. Now *viparīta karaṇī mudrā* is described. It is called the destroyer of multifarious diseases. -120 (b) -122.

Practice of Viparīta Karaṇī Mudrā

nityamabhyāsayuktasya jāṭharāgnivivardhanī /

āhāro bahulastasya sampādyaḥ sādhakasya ca //123//

The digestive fire is increased through the regular practice of *viparīta karaṇī mudra.* Therefore, the *sādhaka* can digest more amount of food. -123.

alpāhāro yadi bhavedagnirdehaṃ haretkśaṇāt /

adhāḥ śiraścordhvapādaḥ kśaṇaṃ syātprathame dine //124//

If the *sādhaka* takes little food, his digestive fire will destroy his body soon. He should raise up his feet keeping the head down for a short time for the first day of his practice. -124.

Result of Viparīta Karaṇī Mudrā

kśaṇācca kiñcidadhikamabhyasettu dinedine /

valī ca palitaṃ caiva ṣaṇmāsārdhānna dṛśyate //125//

Then he should go on increasing the duration of his practice little by little every day. Wrinkles and greying hair (on the body) will not be seen within three to six months. -125.

yāmamātraṃ tu yo nityamabhyasetsa tu kālajit /

vajrolīmabhyasedyastu sa yogī siddhibhājanam //126//

labhyate yadi tasyaiva yogasiddhiḥ kare sthitā /

atītānāgataṃ vetti khecarī ca bhaveddhruvam //127//

He who practices it only for three hours every day, he conquers time. The yogi who practices *vajrolī mudrā* regularly, he is entitled to accomplish *siddhis*. If once he attains *yoga siddhis*, they are ever present at his hands. He knows the past and the future and he certainly can travel in the air. -126-127.

Amarolī Sādhanā

amarīṃ yaḥ pibennityaṃ nasyaṃ kurvandine dine /

vajrolīmabhyasennityamamarolīti kathyate //128//

He who drinks his *amarī* (urine) and draws it in through the nostrils daily and practices *vajrolī* regularly, then it is called a *sādhaka* of *amarolī*. -128.

Perfection in Rāja Yoga

tato bhavedrājayogo nāntarā bhavati dhruvam /

yadā tu rājayogena niṣpanna yogibhiḥ kriyāḥ //129//

Then he is able to accomplish *Rāja Yoga* and certainly there is no doubt about it. When perfection is achieved in *Rāja Yoga*, the yogi does not need any *kriyās* (of *Haṭha Yoga*). -129.

Achievement of Viveka and Vairāgya

tadā vivekavairāgyaṃ jāyate yogino dhruvam /

viṣṇurnāma mahāyogī mahābhūto mahātapāḥ //130//

Then the yogi certainly acquires *viveka* (discrimination) and *vairāgya* (detachment). The God named *Viṣṇu* is indeed *Mahāyogī* (the Great Yogi), *Mahābhūta* (the Great Being) and *Mahātapas* (the Great Ascetic). -130.

Puruṣottama As A Lamp Within

tattvamārge yathā dīpo dṛśyate puruṣottamaḥ /

yaḥ stanaḥ pūrvapītastaṃ niṣpīḍya mudamasnute //131//

Puruṣottama (the Great Personality, i.e. Lord *Viṣṇu*) is seen as a lamp who walk on *tattva mārga* (the path of truth). (This life, having gone through many other lives in the past, comes to human life). The breasts which one suckled (in his earlier life), now enjoys (and experiences) the pleasure by pressing (and playing with) them (in the next stage of life). -131.

Enjoyment of Sensual Pleasure

yasmājjāto bhagātpūrvaṃ tasminneva bhage raman /

yā mātā sā punarbhārya yā bhāryā mātareva hi //132//

The *Jiva* enjoys the pleasure of the same vagina again and again through which he was borne before. One, who was his mother in one birth, will become his wife in next birth (life) and now who is his wife will surely be his mother (in next life). -132.

Cycles of Births with Varied Relations

yaḥ pitā sa punaḥ putro yaḥ putraḥ sa punaḥ pitā /

evaṃ samsāracakreṇa kūpacakre ghaṭā iva //133//

bhramanto yonijanmāni śrutvā lokānsamaśnute /

One who is father will be borne as a son again and one who is son will be born as a father again. In this way, the worldly cycle of death and birth is similar to a bucket of the water-wheel in which the living beings go on wandering constantly through the cycles of deaths and births in varied species and enjoy their worlds. -133-134 (a).

Existence of Three (Vedas, Guṇas, Et Cetera)

trayo lokāstrayo vedāstistraḥ sandhyāstrayaḥ svarāhāḥ //134//

trayo'gnayaśca triguṇāḥ sthitāḥ sarve trayākśare /

trayāṇāmakśarāṇāṃ ca yo'dhite'pyardhamakśaram //135//

There are the three worlds, three *Vedas*, three *sandhyās* (morning, noon and evening), three *svaras* (sounds), three *agnis* and *guṇas* (*sat*, *raj* and *tam*) and they all exist in *trayākśara* (the three alphabets – *A*, *U* and *M*). Therefore, a yogi should study the three alphabets and *ardha akśara* (the half alphabet) as well. -134 (b)-135.

Everything Strung on AUM

tena sarvamidaṃ protaṃ tatsatyaṃ tatparaṃ padam /

puṣpamadhye yathā gandhaḥ payomadhye yathā ghṛtam //136//

tilamadhye yathā tailaṃ pāṣāṇeṣviva kāñcanam /

hṛdi sthāne sthitaṃ padmaṃ tasya vaktramadhomukham //137//

ūrdhvanālamadhobindustasya madhye sthitaṃ manaḥ /

akāre recitaṃ padmamukāreṇaiva bhidyate //138//

makāre labhate nādamardhamātrā tu niścalā /

śuddhasphaṭikasaṅkāśaṃ niṣkalaṃ pāpanāśanam //139//

Everything in this world is strung/inlaid on it. That is the Truth. That is the Supreme Seat. Just like the fragrance in flower, the ghee in milk, the oil in sesame seed and the gold in stones, so everything is pervaded by It. The heart lotus situated in the heart faces downward and its stem is upward. The *bindu* is below it and *mana* (the mind) is situated in the middle of it. Expelled by the breath with the alphabet '*A*', the heart lotus is penetrated with the alphabet '*U*' and *nāda* is attained with the alphabet '*M*'. The *ardhamātrā* (half alphabet) is *niścala* (immovable or silence), like pure crystal, without any parts and destroys all sins. -136-139.

Yoga Means Attaining Liberation – Freedom from Death and Birth

labhate yogayuktātmā puruṣastatparaṃ padam /

kūrmaḥ svapāṇipādādiśiraścātmani dhārayet //140//

evaṃ dvāreṣu sarveṣu vāyupūritarecitaḥ /

niṣiddhaṃ tu navadvāre ūrdhvaṃ prāṅniḥśvasastathā //141//

In this way, the yogi absorbed in yoga attains *parama pada* (the supreme seat, state of liberation). Just like a tortoise pulls in its hands, legs and head (and establishes them within itself), so the inhaled and exhaled *vāyu* through all doors, when the nine gates of the body are closed, starts moving upwards. -140-141.

Ātman Alone Exists

ghaṭamadhye yathā dīpo nivātam kumbhakaṃ viduḥ /

niṣiddhairnavadvārairnirjane nirupadrave //

niścitaṃ tvātmamātreṇāvaśiṣṭaṃ yogasevayetyupaniśat //142//

Just like a lamp kept in the middle of a vessel (has a stable flame), so is the *kumbhaka,* know it. In this yoga *sādhanā* when the nine gates (of the body) are blocked, certainly the pure *ātman* alone remains (in the chamber of the heart) in silence without any disturbances. Thus, here ends the *Yogatattva Upaniśat.* -142.

Śānti Pāṭha

om sahanāvavatu.

saha nau bhunaktu.

saha viryam karavāvahai.

tejasvināvadhītamastu mā vidviśāvahai.

om śāntiḥ   om śāntiḥ om śāntiḥ!

Om. May He protect both of us together. May He nourish both of us together. May both of us get strength and power together. May our knowledge (given and received between us) be powerful. May there be no animosity between us. Om. May there be peace, peace and peace again in all three worlds and May the three types of pains/miseries be peaceful.

KEY TO TRANSLITERATION

Vowels

a ā i ī u ū ṛ ṝ

lṛ lṝ e ai o au aṃ aḥ

Consonants

Gutturals: *ka kha ga gha ṅa*

Palatals: *ca cha ja jha ña*

Cerebrals: *ṭa ṭha ḍa ḍha ṇa*

Dentals: *ta tha da dha na*

Labials: *pa pha ba bha ma*

Semivowels: *ya ra la va*

Sibilants: *śa ṣa sa ha*

Compound Letters: *kṣa tra jña*

Aspirate: *ha*, Anusvara - *ṃ,* Visarga : *ḥ*

Unpronounced *a* - ', *ā* - ''

ABOUT THE AUTHOR

Swami Vishnuswaroop (Thakur Krishna Uprety), B. A. (Majored in English & Economics), received his Diploma in Yogic Studies (First Class) from Bihar Yoga Bharati, Munger, Bihar, India. He was formally trained under the direct guidance and supervision of Swami Niranjanananda Saraswati in the Guru Kula tradition of the Bihar School of Yoga. He was initiated into the lineage of Swami Satyananda Saraswati, the founder of Bihar School of Yoga and the direct disciple of Swami Sivananda Saraswati of Rishikesh. His guru gave his spiritual name 'Vishnuswaroop' while he was initiated into the sannyasa tradition.

Swami Vishnuswaroop is a Life Member of World Yoga Council, International Yoga Federation. Divine Yoga Institute has published his nine books on classical yoga, meditation and tantra. He is one of the few yoga practitioners registered with Nepal Health Professional Council established by The Government of Nepal. He has been teaching on the theory and practice of traditional yoga and the yogic way of life to Nepalese and foreign nationals for more than twenty-five years.

Swami Vishnuswaroop has designed a comprehensive yoga program called 'Yoga Passport' in order to give a broader theoretical and practical knowledge of yoga which includes various aspects of yogic practice. Many health professionals, yoga practitioners and people from various backgrounds of more than forty-seven countries from various parts of the world have gone through his yoga courses and programs. He currently works as the President of Divine Yoga Institute, Kathmandu, Nepal and travels abroad to provide yogic teaching and training.

Made in the USA
Monee, IL
20 July 2020

36730970R00025